DR BARBARA NATURAL SOLUTION FOR INTERSTITIAL CYSTITIS

A Simple Guide to Relief Painful Symptoms through Alkaline, Bladder-Friendly Diet without Negative Effects

KATHONA BODI

CONTENTS

Introduction 7

Getting Started With Dr Barbara Alkaline Diet 10

What Is Interstitial Cystitis? 12

The Role of Diet in IC Treatment 16

Dr Barbara Elimination Diet for IC 18

Additional Tips for Managing Interstitial Cystitis 23

Dr Barbara Alkaline Recipes for IC 26

Conclusion 71

Introduction

Reports show that at least 2-3 percent of men and women in the US are affected by interstitial cystitis. This may not sound like too much but you would be shocked if we were to get into the actual figures. As of 2022, it is estimated that there are over 333.3 million people in the US and this number continues to grow. Now think about what 2-3 percent of 333.3 million looks like. I hope you get it now.

While this might be nothing compared to the prevalence of diabetes, it is definitely something to be worried about. But here is a bigger issue - people who have interstitial cystitis may find it difficult and painful to live with. This is because according to medical science, there is no cure available at the moment.

As a result, a lot of patients often explore alternative solutions to ease the symptoms, and sometimes this might involve keeping to a diet.

The Dr Barbara diet is a plant-based alkaline diet created by a Honduran, late Alfredo Bowman, popularly known as Dr Barbara. According to Dr Barbara, the goal of the diet is to eliminate toxic waste in the body and rejuvenate the cells, and it does this by "alkalizing" the blood.

Since it's vegan, the Dr Barbara diet can be quite restrictive as you will soon discover but that may be what you need to soothe that bladder inflammation.

Getting Started With Dr Barbara Alkaline Diet

As the name suggests, the Dr Sebi diet was developed by Dr Barbara O'Neill, an Australian nutritionist and naturopath who believe in the power of food to heal.

Dr Barbara developed the diet for people who prefer a natural approach to curing diseases or just want to improve their overall health without the use of drugs.

Personally, I like to see it as a maintenance diet, which is important if you want to prevent diseases in the first place.

The whole idea behind the Dr Barbara diet is that disease only exists in an acidic environment. So, the diet aims to make the body more alkaline, which is why it's called an alkaline diet. So, when strictly followed, it promises to detoxify the body and bring it to its natural alkaline state or homeostasis.

According to Dr Barbara, the diet can be used to reverse chronic conditions including lupus, herpes, AIDS, leukaemia and of course, interstitial cystitis.

What Is Interstitial Cystitis?

Interstitial cystitis is a chronic, painful bladder syndrome usually accompanied by pressure and discomfort in the bladder region as well as having the urge to urinate more than usual. It's chronic because it's usually difficult to treat and can constantly reoccur for a long time.

If you found the above definition high-level, you may find this easier to understand:

Do you remember the organs that make up your urinary system? I'm talking about the kidneys, bladder, urethra and ureters.

When someone has interstitial cystitis, their bladder walls become irritated and inflamed. As a result of this irritation and inflammation, you generally feel the need to urinate more often than usual and with a smaller amount of urine.

Women are usually the ones most affected by IC but it can also occur in men and children. As earlier indicated, medically, IC is difficult to treat, although there are medications and therapies that may offer relief.

NB: It is worth mentioning that interstitial cystitis (IC) is not the same as urinary tract infection (UTI) as often mistaken by most people. In IC, there's no infection!

What Causes IC?

The exact cause of IC is not known, however, it's believed that a variety of factors can contribute to the condition.

One of such factors is gender. Like I said earlier, women are the ones more commonly affected by the illness. In fact, nine out of every ten cases diagnosed are usually women.

Another factor is age. People in their 30s or above are more likely to develop IC compared to younger folks.

Likewise, people with a defect in the epithelium of the bladder such as a leak are at higher risk of developing IC. This is because a leaking epithelium makes it easier for toxic waste in the urine to get to the bladder wall, which may cause irritation.

NB: The epithelium is the protective lining of the bladder.

Furthermore, people with chronic pain conditions such as fibromyalgia or IBS have a higher risk of developing interstitial cystitis.

Below are other potential risk factors which can contribute to interstitial cystitis:

- Problem with the pelvic floor muscles
- A UTI that is not diagnosed for a long time
- Immune system inflicted inflammation
- Any damage to the bladder lining

What are the Symptoms?

IC signs are not always the same for every person. Also, it's not uncommon for symptoms to vary over time.

Having said that, here are some common signs and symptoms:

- Urinating frequently, often in very small amounts. This can be up to 50 times a day or even more
- Feeling pain or discomfort in the bladder as it fills. Relief usually comes after urinating.
- (For men) Experiencing pain between the scrotum and anus or perineum
- (For women) Pain in-between the anus and vagina
- Chronic pain in the pelvis
- Constant urge to pee
- You may also experience pain during sexual intercourse

The Role of Diet in IC Treatment

As I mentioned earlier, the exact cause of interstitial cystitis is not clear. Having said that, at its root, the condition is usually associated with the inflammation of the bladder. Now, we all agree that what you eat can have a direct impact on your bladder health.

Consequently, whatever constitutes your meals when you have IC can either minimize the inflammation or make it worse.

With this knowledge, switching to an IC diet such as Dr Barbara Alkaline Diet can be a great way to not only manage IC symptoms but also control flare-ups by addressing it at the root.

Dealing with IC Flare-ups

When you have interstitial cystitis, you may notice that there are certain times when the symptoms are less severe and there are other times you may experience a flare-up. In such situations, some foods can worsen the symptoms or provide relief. As a result, making changes to your diet can be greatly beneficial.

In terms of what food to avoid, studies show that those foods that worsen IC symptoms do so by altering the amount of potassium or pH level of the urine. Some foods may also activate pain receptors in the bladder.

I highly recommend having a dairy where you record your symptoms and what foods you think may be responsible for flare ups; this way, you can avoid such foods in the future.

Dr Barbara Elimination Diet for IC

One of the most natural ways you can treat interstitial cystitis is by following an "elimination diet." From the term, you can easily tell it will involve cutting out certain foods from your diet but it goes beyond that.

It's important to understand that not all IC patients are affected by certain foods the same way. Some people may notice that certain foods tend to worsen their condition.

In fact, studies show that up to 70 percent of people who have IC have had sensitivity to more than one food. Some had greater sensitivity to spicy foods and some kinds of beverages than others. It is also reported that black folks were more sensitive to alcohol and non-caffeinated drinks with more urge to urinate.

Having said, even though a plant-based diet is highly effective for IC, it's still important you figure out your own trigger foods to help relieve you of the symptoms. Once you identify any food, it's better to cut it off for about a week or two; if you notice any decrease in bladder pain, then it means the food is likely contributing to your bladder syndrome. Just to be sure, you can add back the food again and see if it triggers the condition.

Some IC-Friendly Foods

In general, I have found that certain foods can make IC symptoms worse, although the experience might be different for each person.

Some of these include:

- Citrus fruits (some examples include lime, grapefruit, orange and lemon)
- Spicy foods
- Pineapples
- Strawberries
- Caffeine (you will need to limit your caffeine intake or completely avoid it if you discover it's a trigger food for you)
- Carbonated drinks

- Cranberry products (may increase urinary frequency and urgency)
- Tomatoes and other vitamin-C rich foods (if this trigger your symptoms, then I recommend you skip recipes with tomatoes)
- Most acidic foods
- Alcohol
- Condiments
- Artificial sweeteners
- Other beverages such as tea, chocolate and coffee
- Pickled foods
- Processed sandwich meats
- Soy products
- Dairy (limit this or cut it off if it's a trigger; opt for plant-based milk instead)

On the other hand, here's a list of foods that tend to be more IC-friendly:

- Most vegetables, especially leafy greens, root vegetables, and cruciferous vegetables. Common examples are green beans, swiss chard, asparagus, peas, beets, eggplant, spinach, etc

- Gentle beverages; some examples are pear juice, chamomile, and peppermint tea
- Fruits that are low in acidity such as pink lady apple and avocado
- Turmeric and garlic (these help to fight inflammation)
- Fresh fruits such as apricots, pears, papaya, cantaloupe, honeydew, watermelon, etc.
- Whole grains such as brown rice and oats
- Plant-based proteins such as lentils, edamame, broccoli, nuts and seeds, chickpeas, legumes, etc.
- Grain-based coffee substitutes
- Butter from nuts such as cashew, almond, peanut and sunflower
- Nuts such as walnuts, pistachios, cashews, etc.
- Drink a lot of water, up to 6-8 glasses a day, especially if you are not urinating too frequently

Like I said earlier, the easiest way to find out whether any food bothers your bladder is to follow the Dr Barbara Elimination Diet. So, even though you're going plant-based, you still have to be on the lookout for foods that irritate your bladder and cut them out.

In this cases, it might be helpful to keep a food journal where you can record which foods trigger your condition and those that actually improve your bladder health.

While this might take some amount of effort on your path, especially at the initial stages, this will be the best way to create an IC diet intrinsic to your needs.

Additional Tips for Managing Interstitial Cystitis

In addition to following a plant-based diet that is peculiar to your particular situation, there's still certain lifestyle changes you can make that can be very helpful for your condition.

I have listed some of these below:

Reduce Stress

Reduce stress as this will help you better manage the pain. You may need to come up with strategies to deal with emotional and mental stress.

Avoid Smoking

Stop smoking if you do. Smoking can worsen the symptoms.

Avoid Tight Clothing

Avoid wearing tight clothing. Instead opt for something that is loose and more comfortable.

Exercise More

Engage in more physical activities. Some IC-friendly exercises include walking, yoga and Pilates.

Try to Urinate Less

Try to urinate less frequently once you have your bladder pain under control. I can't think of a better way if training yourself to do this than practicing dry fasting. Dry fasting for 12 to 20 hours daily can be very effective if you have a "leaky" bladder.

Try Manipulative Physical Therapy

Some people with pain in their pelvic floor area or tenderness may benefit from manipulative physical therapy.

Practice Intermittent Fasting

Finally, I highly recommend you combine the Dr Barbara Elimination Diet with intermittent fasting for long term benefits.

One of the general requirements of the Dr Barbara Diet is that you have only two meals a day and one light meal. But from a personal experience, I figured out you will get faster results if you reduce your eating to just two meals daily or once (OMAD).

You can have a 6 or 8 hours eating window and fast for the remaining 18 or 16 hours. It's up to you to decide when to eat and when not to eat depending on your schedule. During the time you're fasting, you can have fluids such as water, smoothies or fresh juice, all must be based on a plant-based diet.

In some of my other books, I have a whole chapter dedicated to intermittent fasting.

Dr Barbara Alkaline Recipes for IC

KALE SALAD & HEMP RANCH

Ingredients

- One teaspoon of dill
- Half a teaspoon of sea salt
- Half a cup of hemp seeds
- Two tablespoons of squeezed lime juice
- Half butternut squash, cubed
- Six cups of chopped kale
- Two teaspoons of salt
- One to two tablespoons of grapeseed oil

Instructions

1. Switch on the oven and heat it to up to 350-400 degrees F.
2. Put the hemp seeds, dill, and lime juice in a blender and blend until smooth. You can also use a food processor.

3. Now, toss the kale and squash in the grapeseed oil and add the sea salt. Transfer to a baking dish and roast for 15 to 20 minutes or until cooked. You will know this when the kale gets crispy.

4. Allow to cook, then you can top with dressings.

AVOCADO LETTUCE WRAPS

Ingredients

- One teaspoon of sea salt
- Two avocados, sliced
- One teaspoon of fresh lime juice
- Twelve romaine lettuce leaves
- Two diced bell peppers
- Half red onion (should be diced and sliced)
- Three plum tomatoes, chopped
- One to two teaspoons of cayenne pepper

Instructions

1. Mix all the ingredients in a bowl except the romaine lettuce.
2. Next, you want to wash the lettuce separately. Allow it to dry.
3. Now, place the dry leaves on a plate or dish in such a way that each one forms a natural scoop.

4. Next, pour the mixture you prepared from step one into each leaf so that it fills it. Now, you have your avocado lettuce wraps. Enjoy!

RYE TOMATO & AVOCADO SANDWICH

Ingredients

- Two slices of rye bread
- Two sliced plum tomatoes
- One avocado, sliced
- One to two teaspoons of sea salt
- One to three tablespoons of olive oil
- Half a cup of dandelion greens or purslane

Instructions

1. Place the avocado slices on top of the bread slices.
2. Next, drizzle with olive oil. It should go on top of the avocado.
3. Now, arrange the tomato slices on top of the avocados. You can sprinkle some salt if you wish.
4. Finally, top with purslane. Enjoy your sandwich.

CUCUMBER GAZPACHO

Ingredients

- One avocado, chopped
- Two cups of amaranth greens
- Four plum tomatoes, diced
- Two cucumbers, chopped
- One cup of fresh basil
- Lime juice (prepared from two limes)
- One fennel bulb, chopped with the greens removed
- Half white onion, diced
- One teaspoon of salt
- Olive oil (⅓ cup, can be substituted with avocado oil)

Instructions

1. Start by putting all the ingredients in a food processor or blender. Pulse until smooth.
2. Transfer to jug or any other container of your choice and refrigerate for at least 30 minutes before serving.

SEAWEED SALAD

Ingredients

- Two cups of wakame, chopped (you can also use any other seaweed of your choice)
- ⅔ sliced bell pepper (could be red, yellow or orange)
- Half red/white onion, sliced
- Lime juice prepared from half lime
- Two tablespoons of sesame oil
- Two teaspoons of grated ginger (make sure the ginger is fresh)
- One to two tablespoons of agave nectar

Instructions

1. First soak the seaweed before using it, even if it's not tried. Soak for about 15 minutes or more; this helps with rehydration. After soaking, drain off the water and pat it dry.
2. Next, in a large bowl, combine the seaweed with the other ingredients and stir well to mix.

3. Keep it in the fridge to cool for at least 5 minutes, then serve in smaller bowls or dishes. You can garnish with sesame seeds.

GRANOLA PLATE

Things You Need

- Two and a half cups of oats
- A cup of shredded coconut, unsweetened without preservatives
- 1 tsp of vanilla, extract
- ¾ cup of almonds
- ¼ cup of maple syrup (should be pure)
- ¼ cup of pumpkin seeds
- ½ cup of walnuts (only use if you tolerate it)
- ¼ tsp cinnamon (optional)
- ⅛ tsp of sea salt
- 2 tbsp of coconut oil
- Dried mango to taste (optional, must come without any preservatives)

Cooking Instructions

1. Start by preheating your oven. Set the temperature at 300 degrees Fahrenheit.

2. Transfer the almonds, oats, and walnuts onto cookie sheet.

3. Next, get a small pot and mix the other ingredients - coconut oil, syrup, cinnamon, salt and vanilla. Now pour the mixture on top of the oats and walnuts and flip to mix it up.

4. Then bake for 18-22 minutes. Make sure to stir every 8-10 minutes.

5. When you're done, take it out of the oven, then add the pumpkin seeds and coconut.

6. Bake for an extra 10 to 15 minutes, then take it out and move to a Pyrex dish to get it to cool. Once again, you want to stir often.

7. Optionally, you can cut the dried mango into tiny slices and mix with the granola. Otherwise, skip this step if it's not tolerated. Put it in the fridge to cool.

"MINT" ICED TEA

Things You Need

- 1 tbsp of mint leaves (fresh, ideally should come in a sachet or tea ball)
- Chamomile tea (a bag should be enough)
- 1 teaspoon of sweetener (agave syrup/you can also use raw honey though this is not permitted in Dr Sebi's guide)

Cooking Instructions

1. Get a medium-sized teapot and fill it with water. Now, soak (or steep) the tea for 18-20 minutes.
2. Remove the mint and chamomile. Add your preferred sweetener and stir well. Allow it to cool down, then put it in the fridge.

WATERMELON SALAD

Things You Need

- One red watermelon (small or half-size, seedless)
- One to two cups of English cucumber (sliced)
- Mint sprigs to taste (make sure it's fresh)
- **Blueberries (one half-pint box)**

Cooking Instructions

1. Slice the watermelon into tiny pieces. Next, "scrape off" the outer part, then cut into very small chunks.
2. Transfer the chunks to 1 large bowl or you can divide it into smaller bowls.
3. Next, add the cucumber slices and use the blueberries and sprigs as toppings.

TEFF PORRIDGE

Ingredients

- A pinch of sea salt
- ½ cup teff grain
- 2 cups spring water
- Blueberries to taste (optional)

Instructions

1. Add the water to a saucepan and place over medium/high heat.
2. Bring the water to boil, then add in the teff grain and salt. Stir well.
3. Cover the pan and lower the heat. Simmer for about 15 minutes. Optionally, you can top with a few blueberries.

QUINOA STUFFED MUSHROOMS

Ingredients

- ½ cup quinoa, cooked
- 2 tbsp avocado oil
- ½ tbsp grapeseed oil
- 15 mushrooms, destemmed and scrapped
- ¼ tsp thyme
- 1 plum tomato, diced
- A dash of salt
- ½ tsp walnut, chopped

Instructions

1. Start by preheating the oven at 350°F.
2. Use the avocado oil to brush the mushrooms (should be scrapped first). Then place the mushrooms on a baking sheet and set aside.
3. In a bowl, combine the walnuts, quinoa, grapeseed oil, tomato, thyme and salt.

4. Now fill the mushrooms on the baking sheet with the quinoa stuffing. Bake at 350°F for about 25 minutes. Enjoy!

ELECTRIC SALAD

Ingredients

- 1 cup cherry tomatoes
- 2 red onions
- 1 handful romaine lettuce
- 1 lime (you will need the juice)
- 1 cup kale, chopped
- 3 jalapenos
- Olive oil
- 1 yellow pepper
- 1 orange pepper

Instructions

1. The first thing is to wash and rinse all the ingredients if you have not already done so. Once dry, cut them into smaller pieces.
2. Combine everything in a bowl and drizzle with the lemon juice and oil. Enjoy!

QUINOA PORRIDGE

Ingredients

- ½ tsp cayenne
- ½ lime (you will need to grate the skin)
- 1 cup dry quinoa
- 2 cups water
- ½ cup coconut milk (can be substituted with cream if you wish)
- Cloves to taste
- ½ handful assorted nuts and seeds (optional)

Instructions

1. Prepare the quinoa according to the instructions on the package.
2. After that, pour it into a saucepan (this should be after you have drained the quinoa). Then add the cloves and cayenne. Stir well to combine.
3. Next, add the milk and grated lime (you can also add grated apple if you wish). Stir well to mix.
4. Top with nuts and seeds. Enjoy!

ALKALINE MILLET

Ingredients

- ½ tsp sea salt
- 2 ½ cup water
- 1 cup millet

Instructions

1. The first thing is to dry sauté the millet until golden brown. Then add in the water and salt.
2. Bring the mixture to a boil, then simmer until the water is absorbed. This usually takes about 30 minutes but it could be more depending on the heat.
3. Let everything cool with the lid on. Serve and enjoy!

ZUCCHINI AND HEART MUSHROOM SOUP

Ingredients

- 1 medium zucchini, chopped
- 1 medium-sized onion, chopped (if you eat onion a lot, then you can use a large onion instead)
- 2 bay leaves
- Any vegetable stock of your choice (ideally, homemade)
- 1 tsp grapeseed oil
- 1 lb mushroom, mixed and chopped
- Cayenne pepper to taste
- Sea salt to taste
- Sweet basil to taste

Instructions

1. Start by setting your stove to medium heat. Set a pan with a heavy base on top of the stove, then add the grapeseed oil. Once it gets a little hot, add in the onion and sauté for 5 minutes.

2. Next, add the mushrooms, basil, and bay leaves.
   Allow it to cook for an additional five minutes, then
   add the zucchini. Cook until the vegetables release
   their juices. This might take up to 10-15 minutes.

3. Now, pour in the vegetable stock and bring to a boil.
   Then reduce the heat and simmer for five minutes.

4. Finally, remove the bay leaves from the soup before
   seasoning with salt and pepper. Serve!

MUSHROOM & ONION GRAVY

Ingredients

- 2-3 cups of spring water
- ½ cup mushroom
- 1 tsp sea salt
- ½ cup onion
- ½ tsp oregano
- ¼ cup cayenne
- ½ tsp thyme
- 2 tbsp grapeseed oil
- 3 tbsp garbanzo bean flour
- 1 tsp onion powder

Instructions

1. Start by pouring the grapeseed oil into your frying pan. Then set it on the stove over medium or high heat.
2. Once the oil is a bit hot, add the onion and mushroom and sauté for a minute. Then add the other seasonings and spices, except the cayenne.

3. Sauté for five minutes, then add 2 cups of spring water and the cayenne. Stir well to mix and allow to boil.

4. While you're waiting, sift in the flour little by little, then use a whisk to stir it well in order to reduce lumps.

5. Continue cooking until it boils. You can add more water if you want but don't add not more than one cup. Serve.

GINGER TEA

Ingredients

- 1 pinch cayenne
- 1 thumb fresh ginger root (can be substituted with the powder)
- 4 cups spring water
- 2 tbsp fresh lime juice
- 2 sprigs of new organic dill weed
- Raw agave to taste

Instructions

1. Start by boiling the spring water.
2. While you're waiting, peel the ginger root, then chop it into tiny pieces and add to the boiling water. Also, add the weed.
3. Let it cook for 5 minutes, then strain the tea into a glass jar. Add the lime juice and cayenne and stir.
4. Finally, add the agave to taste. You can have it either hot or cold.

AVOCADO BOWL

Ingredients

- Fresh lime juice from 1 lime
- ½ cup cucumber, chopped
- 2 tbsp melted coconut oil
- 16-20 basil leaves (can be substituted with parsley leaves)
- 1 avocado
- Nuts, chopped
- ⅛ tsp lime zest (you can use more for serving)
- 1 pinch salt
- Agave to taste (optional)

Instructions

1. Start by pouring the lime juice into a blender. Add the avocado and agave. Then blend the mixture until smooth.
2. Now, add the lime zest, cucumber, salt, and coconut oil. Blend again until smooth.

3. Then add the basil or parsley leaves and mix a bit.

4. Transfer to a bowl and top with the chopped nuts.

   You can top with more lime zest if desired.

FRUIT SALAD

Ingredients

- One pint of fresh blueberries
- One ripe pear, cored and diced
- One pint of fresh strawberries, sliced (no stems)
- Two cups grapes, deseeded
- 2 tbsp date syrup (optional)
- ¼ tsp ground cinnamon
- 2 tbsp freshly squeezed lemon juice

Instructions

1. Combine all the ingredients in a bowl. Store in a refrigerator. Serve chill.

HERBERT HUMMUS

Ingredients

- Two garlic cloves
- One cup of fresh basil leaves, blanched and lightly packed
- Four cups of cooked garbanzo beans
- Juice from one lemon
- One cup of vegetable broth
- Half a cup of tarragon leaves, blanched and lightly packed
- Half a cup of fresh, flat parsley leaves
- ¼ cup of chives, chopped
- 2 tbsp sesame seeds, toasted

Instructions

1. Start by dabbing the basil leaves and tarragon until they dry. Now, cut them into smaller bits and put in a blender or food processor.

2. Add in the beans, sesame seeds, lemon juice, garlic, and vegetable broth. Blend until smooth and creamy. Add the chives; stir and serve.

NB: Consume within 4 days.

MISO NOODLE SOUP

Ingredients

- Two scallions, sliced
- One cup of adzuki beans (cooked or canned)
- Four tablespoons of miso
- Two tablespoons of fresh cilantro/basil, chopped
- Seven ounces of soba noodles (100% buckwheat)
- Four cups of water

Instructions

1. Start by pouring some water into a large pot; bring it to a boil.
2. Next, add in the soba noodles and stir. Cook for about five minutes, then drain and rinse (use hot water).
3. In another pot, pour in some water and bring to boil. Remove from heat and add in the miso and stir until dissolved.

4. Finally, add the noodles, adzuki beans, scallions and cilantro to the miso broth. Stir well to combine. Serve warm.

HEMP MILK

Ingredients

- Spring water
- 6 tbsp sea moss gel
- 1 cup hemp seeds

Instructions

1. Start by soaking the hemp seeds in 6 cups of spring water for 30 minutes.
2. Next, transfer the seeds with the water into a blender and blend until smooth.
3. Add in the sea moss and blend for 30 seconds. Store in the refrigerator and use within four days.

TASTY PANINI

Ingredients

- 1 tsp cinnamon
- ¼ cup natural peanut butter
- ¼ cup raisin
- ¼ cup hot water
- Whole grain bread, 2 slices
- 1 ripe banana, peeled and chopped
- 2 tsp cacao powder

Instructions

1. Start by pouring the hot water into a bowl. Add the cinnamon, raisin, and cacao powder and combine.
2. Next, spread the peanut butter on each of the bread slices.
3. Place the chopped banana on the toast.
4. Next, transfer the raisin mixture into a blender and blend until smooth. Spread on the sandwich. Enjoy!

BASIC POLENTA

Ingredients

- One and a half cups of coarse cornmeal
- Five cups of water
- ¾ tsp salt

Instructions

1. Start by pouring the water into a saucepan. Put it on a stove and set to low heat.
2. Gradually add the cornmeal into the water. Then stir until creamy. This might take a couple of minutes.
3. Season with the salt, then transfer the polenta into a bowl. Refrigerate for an hour, then serve.

PECANS & BERRIES SALAD

Ingredients

- Baby arugula or mixed baby greens (15 oz pack)
- Blackberries (half pack, should weigh up to 3 oz)
- Raspberries (half pack, should weigh up to 3 oz)
- Fifteen pecan halves

To make the vinaigrette, here's what you need:

- 3 tbsp extra virgin olive oil
- ⅛ tsp kosher salt
- ⅛ tsp freshly ground pepper to taste
- 1 tbsp champagne vinegar (or rice vinegar/ apple cider vinegar)
- ½ tsp dried basil

Instructions

1. Let's start with the dressing/vinaigrette. Pour the vinegar into a bowl (make sure it's a bowl that won't react with the vinegar). Now add in the basil, pepper, and salt.

2. Next, you want to emulsify the olive oil with the vinaigrette. To do this, drizzle the oil in a slow stream; then whisk together until emulsified.

3. Now, combine the vinaigrette and baby arugula (or mixed greens) and transfer to a salad bowl.

4. Top with pecans, raspberries, and blackberries. Serve immediately.

BUTTERNUT SQUASH SOUP

Ingredients

- One tablespoon of olive oil
- One small onion, chopped
- Two tablespoons of fresh sage, chopped
- Six cups of butternut squash (peeled and cubed, should weigh about 30 oz)
- Half a teaspoon of kosher salt or sea salt
- One sweet apple (ideally, it should be large in size, you will need to peel and chop it)
- Half a teaspoon of cinnamon, grounded
- Half a teaspoon of paprika
- Four and a half cups of vegetable broth
- One tablespoon of fresh ginger, grated
- Half a cup of coconut milk (you can use more for garnish)
- ¼ tsp fresh nutmeg, grated

Instructions

1. Start by preheating your oven to 400 degrees F. Next, mix the apple, sage, squash, cinnamon, onion, paprika, and ¼ tsp salt in a Dutch oven. Toss in one tablespoon of olive oil and combine very well.

2. Roast until the squash becomes tender. This usually takes about half an hour.

3. After that, transfer the Dutch oven to the stove and add in the coconut milk, broth, nutmeg, ginger, and ¼ tsp salt. Allow to boil.

4. Next, you want to blend the mixture. You can either use an immersion blender or you can transfer the soup to the blender in batches. Blend until you get a smooth consistency.

5. When serving, you can drizzle extra coconut milk on top and if you like, add a pinch of nutmeg.

LEMON QUINOA SALAD

Ingredients

- One cup of lentils, cooked
- One cup of quinoa, cooked
- Three tablespoons of olive oil
- One minced garlic clove
- Half a cup of yellow bell pepper, chopped
- Half a cup of red bell pepper, chopped
- ¼ cup freshly squeezed lemon juice
- ¼ cup red onion, chopped
- Salt to taste

Instructions

1. Combine all the ingredients (except salt) in a large bowl. Season with salt to taste.
2. You can season with more grounded pepper if you wish. Serve.

SWEET POTATO & PEANUT CURRY

Ingredients

- A piece of thumb-sized ginger, grated

- 200g bag of spinach

- One tablespoon of coconut oil

- Two cloves of garlic, grated

- One onion, chopped

- One lime, juiced

- 400ml can of coconut milk

- Three tablespoons of Thai red curry paste (ensure it's vegan, you can check for this on the label or packaging)

- One tablespoon of peanut butter

- 500g of sweet potato (after peeling, cut it into small chunks)

- Water

Instructions

1. Start by melting the coconut oil in a saucepan over medium heat. Then add the onion and saute for 4-5 minutes.
2. Next, add in the garlic cloves and ginger and cook for another one minute until the fragrance is released.
3. Now, stir in the other ingredients - curry paste, peanut butter, coconut milk, and sweet potato. Add in about 200 ml of water.
4. Allow the mixture to boil, then reduce the heat and simmer for an additional 20 minutes or until the potatoes become soft. The cover of the saucepan should be removed during this period.
5. Finally, stir in the spinach and lime juice and add your favorite seasoning. Serve alone or with cooked rice (ideally, brown rice or whole grain rice)

MANGO & AVOCADO SALSA

Ingredients

- One garlic clove, minced
- Two tablespoons of fresh lime juice
- One ripe mango (make sure to peel and dice it before use)
- One jalapeno, seeded and diced
- One plum tomato, diced
- One medium Hass avocado, diced
- Half a tablespoon of olive oil
- Two tablespoons of fresh lime juice
- ¼ cup fresh cilantro, chopped
- ¼ cup red onion, chopped
- Pepper and kosher salt to taste

Instructions

1. Mix all the ingredients together in a bowl. Then put it in a refrigerator to marinate for about 30 minutes. Enjoy.

ZUCCHINI & PLUM TOMATOES

Ingredients

- Half a tablespoon of Herbes de Provence (you can find how to make this online)
- One medium-sized zucchini (cut into bits)
- Five medium-sized fresh plum tomatoes, diced
- Two tablespoons of extra virgin olive oil
- Five garlic cloves, smashed
- Fresh pepper and kosher salt to taste

Instructions

1. Pour the olive oil into a large non-stick skillet and heat. Set the stove to medium-high heat.
2. Add in the garlic and sauté until it turns golden. This should take about a minute or two.
3. Now, add in salt and pepper followed by zucchini.
4. Leave it to cook for 4 to 5 minutes on each side. Then introduce the plum tomatoes and Herbes de Provence. You can add additional salt if you desire.
5. Reduce the heat and simmer for 5 to 10 minutes. Serve.

BAKED BANANAS

Ingredients

- 1 banana (ideally, it should be medium ripped; cut it into half lengthwise)
- Half a tablespoon of honey
- Cinnamon to taste

Instructions

1. Start by preheating the oven to 400 degrees F.
2. Arrange the banana halves on a foil or oven-safe dish. Sprinkle with honey and cinnamon.
3. Cover tight with foil, then place it in the oven and allow to bake for 10-15 minutes. Enjoy!
4. Optionally, you can serve with light ice cream or whipped cream.

BUTTERNUT SQUASH LENTIL SOUP

Ingredients

- One bay leaf
- One large onion, diced
- One celery stalk, diced
- One medium-sized carrot, diced
- Half a tablespoon of olive oil
- Six cups of vegetable broth
- Two leeks (we will need only the white part; clean and chop into smaller pieces)
- Two tablespoons of tomato paste
- One pound of butternut, peeled and diced into half inches
- Two ounces of green lentils (this is equivalent to ⅓ cup)
- Three cups of packed chopped lacinato kale (the stems should be removed)
- Half a teaspoon of kosher salt

Instructions

1. Start by heating a Dutch oven or some other heavy pot over medium heat.

2. Once it gets hot, add the olive oil, and follow up with the onions, celery, leeks, and carrots. Reduce the heat and let it cook for 4-5 minutes as you stir it.

3. Now, add in the tomato paste and let it cook for an additional two minutes while stirring.

4. Pour in the vegetable broth, lentils, and bay leaf and allow to boil. Then reduce the heat, cover the pot, and simmer for about 20 minutes.

5. Introduce the butternut and cook until tender. This should take up to 15 minutes or more.

6. Remove the bay leaf, then add salt and pepper as seasoning. Now, add in the kale and allow to cook for 5 to 7 minutes or until the kale becomes tender.

Conclusion

Finally, I hope you found the information in this book useful as you work your way up towards recovery.

Remember, even though a plant-based diet is generally beneficial, each IC case is peculiar and there are still some seemingly healthy foods or ingredients that might trigger your symptoms. You should watch out for these foods and cut down on them when you need to until you've dealt with the problem.

For most IC patients, I have found that citrus fruits (such as lime, lemon, orange and grapefruit) and spicy foods are often a red flag. Also, I recommend you avoid alcohol, caffeine and carbonated drinks. Generally, anything acidic should be avoided as these tend to trigger IC symptoms.

It is also important you consume enough water daily to stay hydrated. Aim to drink 6 to 8 glasses of water each day.